I0757055

Chapter 1: Understanding High-Risk Pregnancies

Definition and Types of High-Risk Pregnancies

High-risk pregnancies are defined as those that carry an increased chance of complications for the mother, the baby, or both. Various factors can elevate the risk level, including pre-existing medical conditions, age, lifestyle choices, and complications that arise during pregnancy. For expecting mothers, understanding the criteria for high-risk classifications is essential to ensure appropriate care and support throughout the pregnancy journey. Women over the age of 35, those with chronic health issues such as diabetes or hypertension, and individuals carrying multiples are commonly classified as high-risk.

There are two primary types of high-risk pregnancies: those that are pre-existing and those that develop during the course of the pregnancy. Pre-existing high-risk pregnancies involve conditions that the mother had before conception, such as autoimmune disorders, heart disease, or severe obesity. These issues require careful management and monitoring from the outset. Conversely, conditions that arise during pregnancy, such as gestational diabetes or preeclampsia, can also categorize a pregnancy as high-risk. The ability to identify these risks early is crucial in managing the health of both mother and child effectively.

Expecting mothers may also encounter lifestyle-related risks that can classify their pregnancy as high-risk. Factors such as smoking, excessive alcohol consumption, and drug use significantly increase the likelihood of complications. Additionally, inadequate nutrition and lack of prenatal care can exacerbate these risks. It is vital for mothers to adopt healthier lifestyles and seek regular medical guidance to mitigate these potential dangers. Understanding these lifestyle factors empowers mothers to make informed choices that benefit their well-being and that of their baby.

In terms of management, high-risk pregnancies often involve more frequent monitoring and specialized care. This can include regular ultrasounds, blood tests, and consultations with specialists such as perinatologists. Expecting mothers may also need to adhere to stricter guidelines regarding physical activity, nutrition, and stress management. Engaging in prenatal fitness and exercise, tailored to individual health needs, can support both physical and mental well-being during this time. It is essential for mothers to communicate openly with their healthcare providers to establish a comprehensive care plan that addresses their specific circumstances.

Lastly, mental health during high-risk pregnancies is a critical aspect that should not be overlooked. The anxiety and stress associated with potential complications can take a toll on an expecting mother's emotional well-being. It is important for mothers to seek support, whether through counseling, support groups, or open conversations with loved ones. Additionally, cultural practices in pregnancy and eco-friendly approaches to childbirth can provide comfort and grounding during this uncertain time. By fostering a supportive environment and prioritizing mental health, mothers can navigate their high-risk pregnancies with greater confidence and resilience.

Common Risk Factors

Understanding the common risk factors associated with high-risk pregnancies is essential for expecting mothers seeking to navigate their journey with knowledge and confidence. High-risk pregnancies can arise from a variety of conditions, which can affect both maternal health and fetal development. Factors such as maternal age, pre-existing medical conditions, and lifestyle choices play a significant role in determining the level of risk. Recognizing these factors early on can empower mothers to take proactive measures to ensure a healthier pregnancy.

Maternal age is one of the most frequently cited risk factors in high-risk pregnancies. Women who are over the age of 35 or under 17 are often considered to be at a higher risk for complications. Advanced maternal age can lead to increased chances of chromosomal abnormalities, gestational diabetes, and hypertensive disorders. Conversely, younger mothers may face risks associated with inadequate prenatal care and higher rates of preterm birth. Awareness of these age-related risks can help mothers make informed decisions regarding their prenatal care and lifestyle adjustments.

Pre-existing medical conditions can significantly impact the course of a pregnancy. Conditions such as diabetes, hypertension, thyroid disorders, and autoimmune diseases can complicate pregnancy and may require specialized management. It is crucial for expecting mothers with these conditions to work closely with their healthcare providers to monitor their health and mitigate potential complications. Adequate management of these health issues can often lead to successful pregnancies and healthier outcomes for both mother and baby.

Lifestyle choices, including nutrition, exercise, and substance use, can also contribute to the risk profile of a pregnancy. Poor dietary habits, lack of physical activity, smoking, and alcohol consumption can all increase the likelihood of complications such as low birth weight, preterm labor, and developmental issues. Expecting mothers should prioritize healthy eating, regular prenatal exercise, and abstaining from harmful substances to enhance their overall well-being. Incorporating eco-friendly practices can further support both maternal and fetal health, aligning with a growing trend towards sustainable living during pregnancy.

Finally, emotional and mental health factors should not be overlooked when assessing risk in pregnancy. Conditions such as anxiety and depression can exacerbate physical health challenges and lead to poor outcomes. Seeking support from mental health professionals, engaging in stress-reducing activities, and fostering a strong support network can significantly improve mental well-being during pregnancy. Understanding and addressing these common risk factors equips expecting mothers with the tools they need to navigate their high-risk pregnancies effectively, promoting a healthier experience for both themselves and their babies.

Importance of Early Detection

Early detection of potential complications during pregnancy is crucial for ensuring the health and well-being of both the mother and the developing fetus. High-risk pregnancies, which may arise due to pre-existing health conditions, age, lifestyle factors, or complications from previous pregnancies, require vigilant monitoring and proactive management. Recognizing warning signs early can lead to timely interventions, which may significantly improve outcomes. Expecting mothers who prioritize early detection are better equipped to navigate the complexities associated with high-risk pregnancies.

Regular prenatal check-ups are essential for early detection. These visits provide an opportunity for healthcare providers to assess the mother's health, monitor fetal development, and conduct necessary screenings. Blood tests, ultrasounds, and other diagnostic tools can reveal potential issues, such as gestational diabetes or preeclampsia, long before they become critical. Expecting mothers should not underestimate the importance of these appointments; they are vital for identifying risks early and formulating appropriate management plans tailored to individual needs.

In addition to medical appointments, self-awareness plays a key role in early detection. Mothers should educate themselves about the signs and symptoms of potential complications. This knowledge empowers them to communicate effectively with their healthcare providers. For instance, understanding the typical patterns of fetal movement can help mothers recognize deviations that may warrant immediate attention. By being attuned to their bodies and the changes they experience, expecting mothers can advocate for their health and the health of their babies.

Mental health is another critical aspect of early detection that should not be overlooked. High-risk pregnancies can lead to increased anxiety and stress, which can affect both the mother and the fetus. Early identification of mental health challenges allows for timely intervention and support, helping mothers cope with the emotional rollercoaster of pregnancy. Resources such as counseling, support groups, and mindfulness practices can be beneficial. Addressing mental health issues early not only fosters a healthier pregnancy but also sets the stage for a positive postpartum experience.

Lastly, the importance of early detection extends beyond the pregnancy itself. It necessitates a holistic approach that considers nutrition, fitness, and family dynamics. Proper nutritional choices and prenatal exercise can mitigate some risks associated with high-risk pregnancies. Furthermore, preparing siblings for a new baby and fostering a supportive environment can enhance family well-being. By recognizing the multifaceted nature of pregnancy and prioritizing early detection, expecting mothers can navigate their high-risk pregnancies more confidently and prepare for a healthier future for themselves and their families.

Chapter 2: Managing Your High-Risk Pregnancy

Regular Prenatal Care

Regular prenatal care is a cornerstone of a healthy pregnancy, particularly for those classified as high-risk. Engaging in consistent prenatal visits allows healthcare providers to monitor both the mother and the developing baby closely. During these appointments, practitioners can conduct necessary screenings, assess vital signs, and address any concerning symptoms or changes. For mothers facing high-risk factors such as advanced maternal age, pre-existing medical conditions, or previous pregnancy complications, the importance of regular check-ups cannot be overstated. These visits provide essential opportunities for early detection and intervention, significantly improving outcomes.

In addition to routine screenings, prenatal care offers an invaluable platform for education and support. Expecting mothers can discuss their concerns, receive guidance on managing their health, and learn about the various stages of pregnancy. This is particularly important for high-risk pregnancies, where tailored advice regarding lifestyle changes, nutrition, and exercise can make a significant difference. Healthcare providers can help mothers develop individualized care plans that incorporate their specific needs, empowering them to take charge of their health and well-being throughout the pregnancy journey.

Nutrition plays a critical role in prenatal care, especially for high-risk pregnancies. Regular consultations with healthcare professionals enable mothers to understand the nutritional requirements essential for sustaining both their health and the baby's development. A well-balanced diet rich in vitamins, minerals, and other nutrients can mitigate some risks associated with high-risk pregnancies. Healthcare providers often recommend specific dietary adjustments, including increased protein intake, proper hydration, and the incorporation of whole foods, to support optimal fetal growth and maternal health.

Mental health during pregnancy is another vital aspect that regular prenatal care addresses. High-risk pregnancies can induce heightened anxiety and stress, which can negatively affect both the mother and baby. Healthcare providers should routinely screen for mental health issues, offering resources and referrals to mental health professionals when necessary. Support groups, counseling, and mindfulness practices can be encouraged during these visits, helping mothers to navigate their emotional well-being while preparing for childbirth.

Finally, regular prenatal care fosters a sense of community and connection for expecting mothers. Meeting with healthcare providers and other mothers creates an environment where shared experiences can be discussed, particularly for those dealing with high-risk circumstances. This sense of belonging can be especially comforting for women who have experienced pregnancy loss or face unique cultural practices. By fostering open dialogue about pregnancy and parenting, regular prenatal visits reinforce the idea that every mother's journey is unique, and support is available to navigate the complexities of bringing a new life into the world.

Monitoring Your Health

Monitoring your health during pregnancy is crucial, especially for those classified as high-risk. Regular check-ups and assessments help ensure that both mother and baby remain healthy throughout the pregnancy journey. Expecting mothers should be proactive in scheduling appointments with their healthcare providers, who will monitor vital signs, growth patterns, and any potential complications. This vigilance is essential in identifying issues early, allowing for timely interventions that can significantly improve outcomes.

Blood pressure monitoring is one of the key components of prenatal care. High blood pressure can lead to serious conditions, such as preeclampsia, which can threaten both maternal and fetal health Expecting mothers should be aware of their baseline blood pressure and report any significant changes to their healthcare provider. Along with blood pressure, regular blood tests can provide valuable insights into the mother's health, including anemia, blood sugar levels, and infections that might impact the pregnancy.

Nutrition also plays a vital role in monitoring health during pregnancy. A well-balanced diet, rich in essential nutrients, can help mitigate some risks associated with high-risk pregnancies. Expecting mothers should focus on consuming a variety of foods, including fruits, vegetables, whole grains, and lean proteins. Additionally, prenatal vitamins are often recommended to ensure that mothers are getting adequate amounts of folic acid, iron, and calcium, which are crucial for fetal development. Keeping a food diary can be an effective way to track dietary intake and identify any deficiencies that may need addressing.

Mental health is equally important during pregnancy, particularly for mothers experiencing high-risk situations. Hormonal changes, coupled with stress related to the pregnancy, can affect emotional well-being. It is essential for expecting mothers to monitor their mental health and seek support when needed. Engaging in mindfulness practices, such as meditation or prenatal yoga, can help alleviate anxiety and promote a sense of calm. Open communication with healthcare providers about mental health concerns can lead to appropriate resources and support systems.

Lastly, introducing eco-friendly practices during pregnancy can contribute to overall health monitoring. Using natural and non-toxic products reduces exposure to harmful chemicals, which can be particularly beneficial for both mother and baby. Expecting mothers should consider incorporating sustainable practices into their prenatal care routines, such as choosing organic foods, using environmentally friendly household products, and minimizing plastic use. By prioritizing both personal health and environmental well-being, mothers can create a nurturing atmosphere for their growing families.

Collaborating with Healthcare Providers

Collaborating with healthcare providers is essential for expecting mothers, especially those facing high-risk pregnancies. Building a strong partnership with your medical team can significantly enhance your pregnancy experience and outcome. It begins with establishing open lines of communication. Discuss your concerns, preferences, and any specific needs you might have. This dialogue not only ensures that you receive personalized care but also helps you feel more empowered and involved in the decision-making process concerning your pregnancy.

Understanding the roles of various healthcare professionals is crucial in fostering effective collaboration. Your primary obstetrician or midwife will guide you through prenatal care, but other specialists may also play vital roles. For example, maternal-fetal medicine specialists focus on high-risk pregnancies, while nutritionists can offer tailored dietary advice. Physical therapists might assist with prenatal fitness, and mental health professionals can support your emotional well-being. Knowing who to turn to for different aspects of your care can help streamline your experience and ensure that all areas of your health are addressed comprehensively.

Equipped with knowledge about your pregnancy and the potential risks involved, you can actively participate in your care plan. This includes asking questions about recommended tests, procedures, and lifestyle adjustments. For mothers interested in natural childbirth, communicating your birth plan and preferences to your team is essential. Providers appreciate when patients articulate their desires, as it fosters a collaborative environment where care can be tailored to fit your values and expectations.

Regular check-ins with your healthcare team can also enhance your collaboration. Schedule routine appointments and follow-up visits to monitor your health and the baby's development. These visits can be opportunities to reassess your birth plan, discuss any changes, and adapt your nutrition and exercise regimens. If you experience any changes in your mental health or emotional well-being, be sure to share this information with your providers. They can offer resources and referrals to help you manage stress or anxiety effectively.

Lastly, consider involving your support system in the collaboration process. Bringing a partner, friend, or family member to appointments can provide additional perspectives and help you remember important information. They can also assist in advocating for your needs, especially if you are feeling overwhelmed. By fostering a cooperative relationship with your healthcare providers and surrounding yourself with supportive individuals, you create a holistic approach to managing your high-risk pregnancy. This not only promotes better health outcomes but also enhances your overall experience during this pivotal time in your life.

Chapter 3: Natural Childbirth Preparation

Understanding Your Options

Navigating a high-risk pregnancy can feel overwhelming, but understanding your options can empower you to make informed decisions about your care. The first step is to familiarize yourself with the classifications of high-risk pregnancies, which can arise from pre-existing medical conditions, complications during pregnancy, or lifestyle factors. By recognizing these categories, you can engage in meaningful conversations with your healthcare provider, ensuring that you receive personalized care that addresses your unique circumstances.

Prenatal care is a cornerstone of managing a high-risk pregnancy. You may need to have more frequent check-ups and specialized tests to monitor the health of both you and your baby. Options such as genetic screening, ultrasounds, and non-stress tests might be recommended to track development and identify potential issues early on. Additionally, engaging in discussions about the possibility of working with a maternal-fetal medicine specialist can provide further insights and tailored support throughout your pregnancy.

Nutrition plays a critical role in the health of both mother and baby, especially in high-risk situations. Understanding your dietary needs is essential for managing complications such as gestational diabetes or hypertension. You should consult a registered dietitian specializing in prenatal nutrition to develop a customized meal plan that focuses on whole foods, adequate hydration, and essential nutrients. Incorporating eco-friendly practices into your diet, like choosing organic produce, can also align with your values while nourishing your body.

Physical fitness is another important consideration during a high-risk pregnancy. Depending on your specific situation, low-impact exercises such as walking, swimming, or prenatal yoga may be beneficial. These activities not only improve your physical well-being but also contribute positively to your mental health. It is crucial to work with your healthcare provider to determine which exercises are safe for you and to develop a routine that supports your overall pregnancy health.

Finally, addressing the emotional aspects of a high-risk pregnancy is vital. The stress and anxiety can be significant, and seeking support through counseling or support groups can be invaluable. Additionally, preparing siblings for the arrival of a new baby and discussing workplace rights regarding maternity leave can alleviate some concerns. By understanding your options in these areas, you can create a comprehensive plan that fosters both your mental well-being and family dynamics, ensuring a smoother transition into motherhood.

Creating a Birth Plan

Creating a birth plan is an essential step for expecting mothers, especially those navigating high-risk pregnancies. A birth plan serves as a roadmap for the labor and delivery experience, outlining your preferences and desires while remaining flexible to the realities of the situation. It is important to view the birth plan as a living document, one that can adapt to changes as necessary, while ensuring that your wishes are communicated effectively to your healthcare team.

When preparing your birth plan, begin by outlining your priorities. Consider aspects such as the environment in which you wish to give birth, your preferences for pain management, and the presence of support people during labor. For mothers with high-risk pregnancies, it is crucial to discuss these elements with your healthcare provider, who can help you understand any limitations or recommendations specific to your situation. This collaboration ensures that your birth plan aligns with medical advice while still reflecting your personal choices.

Incorporate considerations for both natural childbirth preparation and medical interventions into your birth plan. You may wish to express your desire for natural pain relief methods, such as breathing techniques, massage, or hydrotherapy. Conversely, be prepared to make decisions regarding interventions like epidurals, cesarean sections, or the use of forceps if complications arise. Understanding the risks and benefits of each option can empower you to make informed choices that support both your health and your birth experience.

Nutrition and mental health also play significant roles in the lead-up to labor. Include any specific dietary preferences you have during labor and postpartum, especially if you have dietary restrictions or are following an eco-friendly approach to pregnancy. Additionally, consider incorporating strategies for maintaining mental well-being, such as relaxation techniques, affirmations, or even a plan for postpartum support. Having these strategies documented can help ensure that your emotional needs are met during this transformative time.

Finally, ensure that your birth plan takes into account the cultural practices and beliefs that are important to you. If you have specific rituals or traditions that you wish to honor during labor, discuss these with your healthcare provider in advance. Additionally, if you have older siblings, consider how they can be involved in the process, whether through a special role during labor or preparation activities leading up to the arrival of the new baby. By creating a comprehensive birth plan that reflects your values, preferences, and needs, you can foster a sense of control and empowerment throughout your high-risk pregnancy journey.

Techniques for Managing Pain

Managing pain during a high-risk pregnancy can be a complex challenge, but several techniques can help expectant mothers navigate discomfort effectively. Understanding these methods is crucial for both physical and emotional well-being. Pain management strategies can range from natural remedies to medical interventions, and choosing the right approach often depends on individual circumstances, preferences, and the guidance of healthcare providers.

One of the most prominent techniques for managing pain is through prenatal exercise and fitness. Engaging in safe and gentle physical activity can help strengthen muscles, improve flexibility, and increase circulation, all of which contribute to pain relief. Activities such as prenatal yoga or swimming can be particularly beneficial, as they not only reduce discomfort but also promote relaxation and reduce stress. Expecting mothers should consult with their healthcare provider to tailor an exercise routine that aligns with their specific health conditions and pregnancy stage.

Another effective method for pain management is utilizing relaxation techniques. Practices such as deep breathing exercises, meditation, and visualization can help reduce tension and create a sense of calm. These techniques also serve to enhance mental health during pregnancy, helping mothers to cope with anxiety and emotional fluctuations that may arise in high-risk situations. Additionally, incorporating mindfulness into daily routines can promote a greater awareness of the body, encouraging mothers to listen to their needs and respond appropriately.

Natural remedies can also play a role in pain management during pregnancy. Many mothers find relief through herbal teas, essential oils, or acupuncture. For instance, ginger tea is known for its anti-inflammatory properties and can help alleviate nausea and pain. However, it is essential to consult with a healthcare provider before trying any new remedies to ensure safety for both mother and baby. Understanding the potential benefits and risks of natural treatments can empower mothers to make informed decisions regarding their pain management strategies.

Finally, open communication with healthcare providers is vital in developing a personalized pain management plan. Expecting mothers should feel comfortable discussing their pain levels, concerns, and preferences with their doctors or midwives. This collaboration can lead to tailored solutions, including medication options when necessary. Additionally, support groups or counseling can provide emotional support, helping mothers feel less isolated in their experiences and better equipped to manage the challenges of a high-risk pregnancy. By leveraging these techniques, expecting mothers can foster a more positive and empowered pregnancy journey.

Chapter 4: Nutrition and Diet During Pregnancy

Essential Nutrients for High-Risk Pregnancies

Essential nutrients play a crucial role in the health and well-being of both the mother and the developing fetus, particularly in high-risk pregnancies. These pregnancies may involve complications such as gestational diabetes, hypertension, or multiple gestations, making it imperative for expecting mothers to focus on nutrition. A well-balanced diet rich in essential nutrients can help mitigate risks and promote optimal fetal development. It is important for mothers to understand which nutrients are vital during this critical time and how they can incorporate them into their daily meals.

Folic acid is one of the most critical nutrients for pregnant women, especially in high-risk situations. This B-vitamin is essential for the formation of neural tube structures in the developing fetus, which can prevent serious birth defects. Pregnant women should aim for at least 600 micrograms of folic acid daily, and this can be achieved through a combination of supplements and folate-rich foods such as leafy green vegetables, fortified cereals, and legumes. Ensuring adequate folic acid intake not only supports fetal development but also aids in the overall health of the mother, reducing the risk of anemia and other complications.

Iron is another essential nutrient that is particularly significant for those experiencing high-risk pregnancies. Increased blood volume during pregnancy can lead to anemia, which can result in fatigue, weakness, and complications during labor. Pregnant women should aim to consume around 27 milligrams of iron daily. Good sources of iron include lean meats, beans, spinach, and fortified cereals. Pairing iron-rich foods with vitamin C sources, like citrus fruits or bell peppers, can enhance iron absorption, making it an effective strategy to combat potential deficiencies.

Calcium and vitamin D are equally important for both maternal and fetal health. Calcium is necessary for the development of the baby's bones and teeth, while vitamin D plays a role in calcium absorption and supports immune function. Pregnant women should aim for about 1,000 milligrams of calcium and 600 international units of vitamin D each day. Dairy products, fortified plant-based milks, and leafy greens are excellent sources of calcium, while sunlight exposure and fortified foods can help meet vitamin D requirements. Ensuring adequate intake of these nutrients can help prevent complications such as gestational hypertension and support overall pregnancy health.

Lastly, omega-3 fatty acids are vital for brain development and are particularly beneficial during high-risk pregnancies. These healthy fats can help reduce inflammation and may lower the risk of preterm labor. Pregnant women should consider incorporating sources of omega-3s, such as fatty fish, flaxseeds, and walnuts, into their diets. If dietary intake is insufficient, a supplement might be necessary after consulting with a healthcare provider. By prioritizing these essential nutrients, expecting mothers can significantly influence their health outcomes and those of their babies, fostering a healthier pregnancy journey.

Meal Planning and Preparation

Meal planning and preparation during a high-risk pregnancy is an essential aspect of maintaining both maternal and fetal health. For expecting mothers, understanding the importance of nutrition can significantly impact the outcomes of their pregnancies, especially when faced with additional challenges. A well-thought-out meal plan not only ensures that the mother receives the necessary nutrients but also helps mitigate stress and anxiety surrounding food choices. It involves selecting wholesome ingredients, creating balanced meals, and setting aside time for cooking, which can be especially beneficial for those managing high-risk pregnancies.

When planning meals, it is crucial to focus on a variety of food groups to ensure adequate intake of vitamins and minerals. This includes incorporating lean proteins, whole grains, healthy fats, fruits, and vegetables into daily diets. Foods rich in folate, iron, calcium, and omega-3 fatty acids are particularly important, as they support fetal development and maternal health. Expecting mothers should consider working with a registered dietitian who specializes in prenatal nutrition to create personalized meal plans that align with their specific health needs and dietary restrictions.

Preparation plays a significant role in making meal planning manageable. Setting aside a few hours each week for meal prep can ease daily cooking burdens, allowing mothers to focus on their health and well-being. Batch cooking and freezing meals can provide quick, nutritious options during busy days or when fatigue sets in. Simple recipes that require minimal ingredients and time can help maintain a healthy diet without overwhelming the mother, reinforcing the idea that nutritious meals do not have to be complex or time-consuming.

In addition to physical nutrition, meal planning can also address emotional well-being. Engaging in a structured approach to meals can foster a sense of control and routine, which is beneficial for mental health during pregnancy. For mothers navigating the emotional landscape of a high-risk pregnancy, creating a meal plan can serve as a grounding practice, allowing them to focus on nourishing their bodies and their babies. Sharing meals with family members can also strengthen bonds and provide support, making mealtime an opportunity for connection.

Finally, considering eco-friendly practices in meal planning and preparation can further enhance the experience. Choosing locally sourced, organic ingredients not only supports sustainable agriculture but also reduces exposure to harmful chemicals. Additionally, meal planning can incorporate cultural practices and traditions, allowing mothers to celebrate their heritage while ensuring nutritional needs are met. By combining health-focused meal planning with environmental consciousness and cultural appreciation, expecting mothers can create a supportive and enriching environment for themselves and their growing families.

Safe Foods and Foods to Avoid

Safe foods during pregnancy are crucial for the health of both the mother and the developing baby. Foods that are rich in essential nutrients, such as fruits, vegetables, whole grains, lean proteins, and healthy fats, should form the foundation of a pregnant woman's diet. Fresh fruits and vegetables provide vital vitamins and minerals, while whole grains like brown rice and quinoa offer necessary fiber that aids digestion and helps prevent gestational diabetes. Lean proteins, including poultry, fish, beans, and legumes, are essential for the growth and development of the fetus. Healthy fats, particularly those from sources like avocados, nuts, and olive oil, support brain development and overall health.

Certain foods are particularly beneficial during a high-risk pregnancy. Foods high in folate, such as leafy greens, fortified cereals, and citrus fruits, can reduce the risk of neural tube defects. Omega-3 fatty acids, found in fatty fish like salmon and walnuts, play a significant role in fetal brain development. It is also important to include calcium-rich foods like dairy products, almonds, and fortified plant-based alternatives to support the growing baby's bones and teeth. Staying hydrated with plenty of water is equally vital, as it helps maintain amniotic fluid levels and supports overall health.

Conversely, there are foods that expecting mothers should avoid to reduce the risk of complications. Raw or undercooked meats, eggs, and seafood can harbor harmful bacteria and parasites. Pregnant women should also steer clear of unpasteurized dairy products and juices, as they can pose a risk of foodborne illnesses. Certain fish, particularly those high in mercury like shark, swordfish, and king mackerel, should be limited due to potential neurological risks to the developing fetus. Additionally, processed foods high in sugar, salt, and unhealthy fats can contribute to excessive weight gain and other complications during pregnancy.

Caffeine and alcohol consumption should also be carefully considered. High caffeine intake has been linked to an increased risk of miscarriage and low birth weight, so many health professionals recommend limiting caffeine to about 200 milligrams a day, roughly equivalent to one 12-ounce cup of coffee. Alcohol, on the other hand, is best avoided entirely, as there is no known safe amount during pregnancy, and its effects on fetal development can be severe, leading to fetal alcohol spectrum disorders.

Finally, it's essential to approach dietary changes with mindfulness and awareness of individual health conditions and cultural practices. Pregnant women should consult with healthcare providers or nutritionists to tailor their diets according to their specific needs, especially in high-risk situations. Understanding cultural dietary practices can also play a significant role in creating a balanced diet that respects heritage while promoting health. By focusing on safe foods and being aware of those to avoid, expecting mothers can take proactive steps to ensure a healthy pregnancy for themselves and their babies.

Chapter 5: Prenatal Fitness and Exercise

Benefits of Exercise During Pregnancy

Exercise during pregnancy offers numerous benefits that can significantly enhance the overall well-being of expecting mothers, especially those navigating high-risk pregnancies. Engaging in regular physical activity can help manage weight gain, reduce the risk of gestational diabetes, and improve cardiovascular health. For mothers who may be concerned about their health or the health of their developing baby, maintaining a consistent exercise regimen can provide a sense of control and empowerment during a time that may often feel overwhelming.

Moreover, prenatal exercise has been shown to alleviate common pregnancy-related discomforts such as back pain, fatigue, and swelling. Activities like walking, swimming, and prenatal yoga can promote better posture and flexibility, which can be particularly beneficial as the body changes and adapts to accommodate the growing baby. This physical preparation can not only improve comfort levels but also enhance the body's ability to cope with the physical demands of labor and childbirth.

In addition to physical benefits, exercise has a positive impact on mental health during pregnancy. Engaging in regular physical activity can help combat anxiety and depression, which are not uncommon among expecting mothers, particularly those facing complications or high-risk factors. The release of endorphins during exercise contributes to improved mood and reduced stress levels. This emotional resilience is vital for mothers as they prepare for the challenges of childbirth and parenthood.

Another significant advantage of exercising during pregnancy is the potential for better birth outcomes. Research indicates that women who maintain an appropriate fitness routine are more likely to experience shorter labor, fewer complications, and a lower likelihood of needing interventions such as cesarean sections.

Furthermore, these women often report higher satisfaction levels with their birthing experience, which can positively influence their transition into motherhood.

Finally, prenatal fitness can also foster a supportive community among expecting mothers. Participating in group classes or activities can create a network of social support, essential for emotional well-being. Building connections with others who share similar experiences can help alleviate feelings of isolation and promote a sense of belonging during this transformative period. As mothers prepare for the arrival of their newborns, the benefits of exercise extend beyond physical health, enriching their mental and emotional journey as well.

Safe Exercises for High-Risk Pregnancies

Engaging in physical activity during pregnancy can be beneficial, even in high-risk situations, but it is essential to choose exercises that prioritize safety and comfort. High-risk pregnancies may involve complications such as gestational diabetes, hypertension, or a history of preterm labor. Therefore, expecting mothers must consult with their healthcare providers to develop a tailored exercise plan that considers their specific circumstances. Low-impact exercises are generally recommended, as they minimize the risk of injury while promoting physical well-being.

Walking is one of the safest and most accessible forms of exercise for pregnant women. It can be easily adjusted in terms of intensity and duration, making it suitable for various fitness levels. Walking not only helps maintain cardiovascular health but also improves mood and energy levels. Pregnant women should aim for moderate walking, which can be done in short sessions throughout the day to accommodate any fatigue or discomfort. Wearing supportive footwear can further enhance comfort during these walks.

Swimming is another excellent option for high-risk pregnancies, as it provides a full-body workout without the strain of gravity. Water exercise can relieve pressure on joints and reduce swelling, making it particularly beneficial for those experiencing discomfort. Swimming also allows for improved circulation and can help regulate body temperature. Expecting mothers should consider joining specialized water aerobics classes for pregnant women, which focus on safe techniques and exercises designed to strengthen the body while minimizing risks.

Prenatal yoga is a valuable practice that combines gentle stretching, breathing techniques, and relaxation methods. It can help alleviate anxiety and stress, which are common during high-risk pregnancies. Specific poses can improve flexibility and strength while enhancing mental well-being. However, it is crucial to choose classes led by certified instructors experienced in prenatal yoga to ensure that the exercises are safe and appropriate for each stage of pregnancy. Modifications can be made to accommodate any physical limitations.

Finally, incorporating pelvic floor exercises, such as Kegel exercises, can be particularly beneficial during pregnancy. Strengthening the pelvic floor can help prepare the body for labor and delivery while also aiding in recovery postpartum. These exercises can be performed discreetly throughout the day and provide long-term benefits, including improved bladder control. Expecting mothers should always discuss their exercise choices with their healthcare providers to ensure that they align with their overall health and pregnancy goals. By prioritizing safe exercises, mothers can support their health and well-being during this crucial time.

Creating a Fitness Routine

Creating a fitness routine during pregnancy is essential for maintaining overall health and well-being, especially for expecting mothers navigating high-risk pregnancies. A well-structured fitness plan can help manage physical discomfort, improve mood, and enhance overall pregnancy outcomes. It is important to consult with healthcare providers before starting any exercise program, particularly for those with specific medical conditions or concerns. A personalized approach that considers individual health status and lifestyle is crucial in developing an effective routine.

When designing a fitness routine, it is beneficial to incorporate a variety of exercises to ensure a balanced approach. Low-impact activities such as walking, swimming, and stationary cycling are excellent choices for most expecting mothers, as they minimize stress on the joints while providing cardiovascular benefits. Additionally, strength training with light weights or resistance bands can help maintain muscle tone and improve endurance. Flexibility exercises, such as prenatal yoga or gentle stretching, should also be included to enhance mobility and reduce tension in the body.

The frequency and duration of workouts should be adjusted according to each mother's comfort level and energy. Generally, engaging in moderate exercise for at least 150 minutes a week is recommended, which can be broken down into manageable sessions throughout the week. It is important to listen to the body and make modifications as needed. If fatigue or discomfort arises, it may be wise to reduce the intensity or duration of workouts. Hydration and proper nutrition are equally vital components that support an active lifestyle during pregnancy.

In addition to the physical benefits, establishing a fitness routine can significantly enhance mental health during pregnancy. Regular exercise releases endorphins, which can help alleviate feelings of anxiety and depression. Participating in group classes or prenatal exercise programs can also foster a sense of community among expecting mothers, providing emotional support and shared experiences. Mindfulness practices, such as meditation or focused breathing incorporated into a fitness routine, can further promote relaxation and a positive mindset.

Lastly, it is essential to recognize the importance of adaptability in a fitness routine, especially for those experiencing high-risk pregnancies. As pregnancy progresses, physical limitations may arise, and it is vital to remain flexible and make necessary adjustments. Engaging with healthcare professionals to monitor progress and discuss any concerns can ensure safety and effectiveness. By prioritizing a well-rounded fitness routine, expecting mothers can take proactive steps toward a healthier pregnancy experience while fostering resilience in the face of challenges.

Chapter 6: Mental Health During Pregnancy

Recognizing Mental Health Challenges

Recognizing mental health challenges during pregnancy is crucial for the well-being of both the mother and the developing baby. Pregnancy, particularly high-risk pregnancy, can be an emotionally charged experience, often leading to feelings of anxiety, depression, or stress. It is vital for expecting mothers to understand that these feelings are not uncommon and that recognizing them early can lead to better outcomes. Awareness of one's mental health is the first step toward effective management and support.

Common mental health challenges include prenatal anxiety, which may manifest as excessive worrying about the pregnancy, the health of the baby, or the upcoming labor and delivery. Additionally, some mothers may experience prenatal depression, characterized by persistent sadness, loss of interest in activities, and difficulty bonding with the unborn child. Recognizing these symptoms can help mothers seek help before they escalate. It's important to note that these feelings can be exacerbated by the stresses associated with high-risk pregnancies, such as medical complications or previous pregnancy losses.

Expecting mothers should also be aware of the impact of hormonal changes on mental health during pregnancy. Fluctuations in hormones can lead to mood swings and heightened emotional sensitivity. Additionally, the physical changes associated with pregnancy can affect self-esteem and body image, further contributing to mental health struggles. Understanding these changes allows mothers to anticipate potential difficulties and seek support from healthcare providers or mental health professionals.

Cultivating a strong support system is essential in recognizing and addressing mental health challenges. Engaging with family, friends, and healthcare providers can provide emotional reassurance and practical assistance. Participating in prenatal classes or support groups can also foster connections with other expecting mothers who may share similar experiences. These connections can help reduce feelings of isolation and provide a platform for discussing mental health openly.

Lastly, expecting mothers should prioritize self-care and mental wellness as part of their overall pregnancy plan. This includes maintaining a balanced diet, engaging in regular physical activity, and practicing relaxation techniques, such as mindfulness or meditation. Additionally, understanding workplace rights can ensure that mothers receive the necessary accommodations to maintain their mental health during pregnancy. By recognizing the signs of mental health challenges and actively seeking support, expecting mothers can navigate their high-risk pregnancies with greater confidence and resilience.

Coping Strategies and Support Systems

Coping strategies and support systems play a critical role in managing the complexities of high-risk pregnancies. Expecting mothers facing such circumstances often experience heightened anxiety and emotional strain. It is essential for these mothers to develop personalized coping strategies that can be integrated into their daily lives. Techniques such as mindfulness, deep breathing exercises, and journaling can help alleviate stress and promote mental clarity. Additionally, maintaining a structured routine can provide a sense of normalcy, which is particularly beneficial during unpredictable pregnancy journeys.

Support systems are equally vital in navigating the challenges of high-risk pregnancies. Engaging with family, friends, and healthcare providers can create a robust network that reinforces emotional and practical support. Mothers should not hesitate to share their feelings and concerns with loved ones, as this can foster understanding and encouragement. Moreover, joining support groups, either in-person or online, allows for the sharing of experiences and strategies with others facing similar situations, helping to combat feelings of isolation.

Professional support is another cornerstone of effective coping strategies. Regular consultations with healthcare providers enable expecting mothers to stay informed about their health and any necessary precautions. Mental health professionals can also provide therapy or counseling tailored to the unique stresses of high-risk pregnancies. Recognizing when to seek help is crucial, as mental well-being directly influences physical health during this critical time. Accessing counseling services can equip mothers with additional tools to manage anxiety and depression.

Incorporating nutrition and fitness into a high-risk pregnancy plan can also serve as beneficial coping strategies. A balanced diet rich in essential nutrients supports both maternal and fetal health, fostering a sense of agency over one's body. Likewise, prenatal exercise, under professional guidance, can enhance physical strength and mental resilience. Activities such as gentle yoga or walking can elevate mood, improve sleep quality, and reduce stress, contributing to a more positive pregnancy experience.

Finally, addressing workplace rights and preparing siblings for a new baby are essential elements of a comprehensive support system. Expecting mothers should familiarize themselves with their rights regarding maternity leave and workplace accommodations, ensuring they can advocate for themselves effectively. Additionally, preparing siblings for the arrival of a new baby can help ease family transitions and reduce anxiety. Engaging children in discussions about the pregnancy, using books or activities that explain the process, can foster excitement rather than apprehension, creating a cohesive family unit ready to welcome the new addition.

When to Seek Professional Help

Recognizing when to seek professional help during a high-risk pregnancy is crucial for the health and well-being of both the mother and the baby. High-risk pregnancies can arise from a variety of factors, including pre-existing medical conditions, age, lifestyle choices, and complications that develop during pregnancy. Expecting mothers should be aware of specific warning signs and symptoms that warrant immediate medical attention, such as severe abdominal pain, heavy bleeding, or sudden swelling of the hands and feet. These indicators can signal potential complications that, if addressed promptly, can significantly improve outcomes for both mother and child.

In addition to obvious physical symptoms, mental health is an essential aspect of pregnancy that should not be overlooked. Many expecting mothers experience anxiety, depression, or stress, which can be exacerbated by the uncertainties associated with a high-risk pregnancy. It is important for mothers to recognize when their emotional well-being is being compromised. Seeking help from a mental health professional or a support group can provide vital coping strategies and reassurance, allowing mothers to navigate their pregnancy with greater confidence and peace of mind.

Expecting mothers should also consider seeking professional help if they have questions or concerns about their nutrition and diet during pregnancy, particularly in high-risk situations. A registered dietitian or nutritionist specializing in prenatal care can offer personalized dietary advice that meets the unique needs of high-risk pregnancies. This guidance can help ensure that mothers receive adequate nutrition, which is essential for fetal development and can mitigate some risks associated with complicated pregnancies.

Regular prenatal check-ups are vital for monitoring the health of both mother and baby, but there are certain circumstances that may require more frequent or specialized care. If an expecting mother has experienced a previous pregnancy loss, she may benefit from additional emotional and medical support. Healthcare providers can offer tailored monitoring and interventions, which can help address any underlying issues and provide a more reassuring experience during subsequent pregnancies.

Finally, it is essential for expecting mothers to advocate for themselves and understand their rights in the workplace, especially during a high-risk pregnancy. Knowing when to seek professional help can also extend to legal advice regarding workplace accommodations, maternity leave, and any other concerns related to their employment status. Engaging with professionals who understand the complexities of maternal rights can empower mothers to take the necessary steps to ensure their health and the health of their unborn child are prioritized during this critical time.

Chapter 7: Pregnancy After Loss

Navigating Grief and Healing

Grief is a complex and deeply personal experience, especially for expecting mothers navigating high-risk pregnancies. The anticipation of bringing a new life into the world can be overshadowed by anxiety, loss, or uncertainty, particularly if there have been previous pregnancy losses or complications. Understanding the multifaceted nature of grief during this sensitive time is crucial. Recognizing that it is normal to experience a range of emotions—sadness, anger, guilt, or even moments of joy—can help mothers process their feelings and begin the journey toward healing.

Healing from grief does not follow a linear path; it is often filled with ups and downs. For mothers facing high-risk pregnancies, the pressure to maintain a positive outlook may be overwhelming. It is important to prioritize mental health, seeking support through counseling, support groups, or talking openly with trusted family and friends. Engaging in mindfulness practices, such as meditation or gentle yoga, can also provide a sense of calm and clarity, allowing mothers to confront their emotions healthily and constructively.

Creating a safe space for emotions is vital in navigating grief. This can involve journaling, expressing feelings through art, or even engaging in conversations with other mothers who have experienced similar challenges. It is essential to honor personal grief and recognize that healing is unique to each individual. Some mothers may find solace in rituals or ceremonies that acknowledge their loss, while others might prefer to focus on the present and future. Finding what resonates personally can facilitate a deeper understanding of one's feelings and contribute to emotional resilience.

Physical health plays an integral role in emotional well-being during this time. Maintaining a balanced diet rich in nutrients can help stabilize mood and energy levels. Incorporating prenatal exercise, tailored to individual capabilities and doctor recommendations, can also promote mental well-being. Activities such as walking, swimming, or prenatal yoga not only support physical health but can also serve as an outlet for stress relief. Staying active helps in the release of endorphins, which are natural mood enhancers, contributing to a more positive outlook.

Finally, it is essential for expecting mothers to seek out community and connection. Sharing experiences with others who understand the challenges of high-risk pregnancies can foster a sense of belonging and reduce feelings of isolation. Online forums, local support groups, or classes focused on pregnancy after loss can provide invaluable resources and encouragement. By building a supportive network, mothers can navigate their grief while preparing for the new life they are bringing into the world, creating a balanced approach to both healing and anticipation.

Preparing for a New Pregnancy

Preparing for a new pregnancy is a multifaceted journey that requires careful consideration and planning, especially for those with a history of high-risk pregnancies. The first step in this process involves a thorough medical consultation to assess your individual health status. Engaging with healthcare providers who specialize in high-risk pregnancies can provide valuable insights into your specific needs and potential challenges. Understanding your medical history, any previous pregnancy complications, and current health conditions will help establish a tailored plan that prioritizes your well-being and that of your future child.

Nutrition plays a vital role in preparing for pregnancy, particularly for those with heightened risks. A balanced diet rich in essential nutrients supports overall health and can help mitigate some risks associated with pregnancy. Focus on consuming a variety of fruits, vegetables, whole grains, and lean proteins. Additionally, consider consulting a nutritionist to create a personalized meal plan that aligns with your dietary needs and goals. Supplements such as folic acid are crucial in the preconception phase to reduce the risk of neural tube defects. Ensuring that your body is nourished adequately before conception can set a positive foundation for a new pregnancy.

Physical fitness is another critical component of preparation. Engaging in regular prenatal exercise not only enhances physical strength and stamina but also promotes mental well-being. Activities such as walking, swimming, and prenatal yoga can be beneficial, especially for women with high-risk factors. Always consult your healthcare provider before starting any exercise regimen to ensure that the activities are safe and appropriate for your situation. Establishing a consistent fitness routine will help you build resilience and prepare your body for the demands of pregnancy and childbirth.

Mental health is equally important when preparing for a new pregnancy, particularly for those who have experienced loss or previous complications. It is essential to address any emotional concerns and seek support from mental health professionals if needed. Building a strong support network of family, friends, or support groups can provide comfort and reassurance. Mindfulness practices, such as meditation and deep-breathing exercises, can also help manage anxiety and stress during this transitional phase. Prioritizing your mental health is vital in fostering a positive environment for yourself and your future baby.

Lastly, consider the implications of this new pregnancy on your existing family dynamics, especially if you have other children. Preparing siblings for a new baby involves open communication and involvement. Share the excitement of the upcoming addition and encourage them to express their feelings about the change. Engaging them in the preparation process, such as choosing baby clothes or decorating the nursery, can foster a sense of inclusion and excitement. Additionally, educate yourself on workplace rights to ensure you can navigate any necessary adjustments during your pregnancy, allowing you to focus on what truly matters: welcoming your new child into a supportive and loving environment.

Building a Support Network

Building a support network is an essential step for expecting mothers, particularly those navigating high-risk pregnancies. The emotional and physical challenges that accompany a high-risk status can feel overwhelming, making it crucial to surround yourself with individuals who can provide understanding, encouragement, and practical assistance. This network should include family, friends, healthcare professionals, and support groups that resonate with your unique circumstances. Each member plays a vital role in ensuring you feel supported throughout your pregnancy journey.

Family and friends often form the backbone of your support network. They can offer emotional reassurance, help with daily tasks, and provide companionship during medical appointments. Open communication about your needs and feelings is key. Let them know how they can assist you, whether it's through attending prenatal classes, accompanying you to doctor visits, or simply being there to listen when you need to talk. Remember that your loved ones may also need guidance on how to best support you, so sharing your experiences can foster understanding and strengthen these relationships.

Healthcare professionals are another critical component of your support network. Establishing a trusting relationship with your obstetrician, midwife, and any specialists involved in your care can empower you to make informed decisions about your pregnancy. Don't hesitate to ask questions or express concerns during appointments. Additionally, consider reaching out to a prenatal nutritionist or fitness expert who specializes in high-risk pregnancies. Their expertise can help you create a personalized plan that addresses your dietary needs and fitness goals while keeping your safety at the forefront.

Support groups can also provide a sense of community and understanding that may be hard to find elsewhere. These groups often consist of other expecting mothers who are facing similar challenges. Sharing experiences and advice can be incredibly beneficial, allowing you to feel less isolated in your journey. Look for local or online support groups dedicated to high-risk pregnancies, pregnancy after loss, or even eco-friendly pregnancy practices. Engaging with others who share your interests and concerns can foster a sense of belonging and emotional relief.

In addition to these traditional forms of support, consider the importance of mental health during pregnancy. Seeking help from a therapist or counselor who specializes in prenatal mental health can be invaluable, especially if you're feeling anxious or overwhelmed. They can provide coping strategies tailored to your situation, helping you to manage stress and maintain a positive mindset. Ultimately, a well-rounded support network that encompasses emotional, physical, and informational resources will empower you to navigate your high-risk pregnancy with confidence and resilience.

Chapter 8: Eco-Friendly Pregnancy and Parenting

Sustainable Choices During Pregnancy

Sustainable choices during pregnancy are increasingly recognized as beneficial not only for the expecting mother but also for the environment and future generations. As women navigate the complexities of high-risk pregnancies, making environmentally conscious decisions can contribute positively to their overall well-being. This subchapter will explore practical ways expecting mothers can embrace sustainability through various aspects of their pregnancy journey, including nutrition, fitness, and mental health.

Nutrition plays a vital role in high-risk pregnancies, and choosing organic, locally sourced foods can significantly impact both maternal health and environmental sustainability. Organic foods are often free from harmful pesticides and chemicals, which is particularly important during pregnancy when developing fetuses are more vulnerable. By opting for seasonal produce from local farmers' markets, expecting mothers can reduce their carbon footprint while ensuring they receive fresh, nutrient-dense foods. Additionally, incorporating plant-based meals can lower the environmental impact of one's diet, promoting better health outcomes for both mother and baby.

Prenatal fitness and exercise are crucial components of a healthy pregnancy, and sustainable practices can enhance this experience. Expecting mothers can engage in eco-friendly activities such as yoga or walking in nature, which not only promote physical health but also foster a connection with the environment. Choosing to participate in classes that emphasize sustainability, such as those that use natural materials or support local communities, can further enrich the prenatal fitness experience. Additionally, incorporating mindful practices like meditation can help alleviate stress, contributing to improved mental health during this critical time.

Mental health is a priority during pregnancy, and sustainable choices can extend to emotional well-being. Engaging with support groups that focus on eco-friendly parenting can provide a sense of community and shared values among expecting mothers. These groups often emphasize natural childbirth preparation and eco-conscious parenting practices, creating a supportive network that nurtures both mental and physical health. Furthermore, integrating sustainable practices into daily routines, such as minimizing waste and reducing plastic use, can foster a sense of purpose and empowerment, which is particularly beneficial for mental wellness during high-risk pregnancies.

Cultural practices surrounding pregnancy can also incorporate sustainable choices, allowing expecting mothers to honor their traditions while promoting environmental consciousness. Many cultures celebrate pregnancy through rituals and practices that can be adapted to align with eco-friendly values. For instance, using natural materials for ceremonies or gifting locally made items can enhance the cultural experience while supporting local artisans. By blending sustainable practices with cultural traditions, mothers can create a nurturing environment that honors both their heritage and their commitment to the planet, ultimately setting a positive example for their children.

Eco-Friendly Baby Products

The increasing awareness of environmental issues has led many expecting mothers to seek eco-friendly baby products as part of their preparation for a new arrival. Eco-friendly baby products are designed with sustainability in mind, often made from organic, biodegradable, or recycled materials that minimize the impact on the planet. When selecting these products, mothers can make choices that not only safeguard their child's health but also contribute to a healthier environment. For mothers managing high-risk pregnancies, choosing non-toxic and chemical-free options can be particularly crucial, as exposure to harmful substances may pose additional risks.

One of the most significant categories of eco-friendly baby products includes clothing and textiles. Organic cotton baby clothes are a popular choice, as they are free from harmful pesticides and chemicals used in conventional cotton farming. Additionally, many brands now offer bamboo or hemp clothing, which are not only sustainable but also hypoallergenic and incredibly soft for a baby's sensitive skin. Using eco-friendly laundry detergents is also essential; these products are typically made from plant-based ingredients that are gentle on both the skin and the environment, making them suitable for newborns.

In the realm of baby gear, expecting mothers can find a variety of eco-friendly options ranging from cribs to strollers. Many manufacturers are now creating furniture from sustainably sourced wood and using non-toxic finishes to ensure safety. Strollers and carriers made from recycled materials or organic fabrics are also available, providing safe and durable options for mobility. These products not only support the health of the child but also reflect a commitment to sustainability that can set a positive example for future generations.

When it comes to feeding, eco-friendly baby products include reusable cloth diapers and organic baby food. Cloth diapers reduce waste significantly compared to disposables and are often made from natural fibers, which are gentler on the baby's skin. Organic baby food, available in jars or pouches, is made from fruits and vegetables free from pesticides and artificial additives. This choice not only nurtures the infant's developing system but also promotes a healthy lifestyle that can continue as the child grows.

Lastly, the importance of mental health during pregnancy cannot be overstated, and choosing eco-friendly products can contribute positively to an expecting mother's well-being. The act of making thoughtful and sustainable choices can foster a sense of empowerment and connection to the planet. Additionally, engaging in practices that promote eco-consciousness can serve as a calming ritual, offering a sense of purpose and mindfulness during what can be a stressful time. By integrating eco-friendly baby products into their lives, expecting mothers not only prepare for their child's arrival but also embrace a lifestyle that prioritizes health, sustainability, and well-being.

Raising an Environmentally Conscious Child

Raising an environmentally conscious child begins even before birth, especially for expecting mothers navigating high-risk pregnancies. It is essential to create a nurturing environment that emphasizes sustainability and awareness of ecological issues. This foundational approach can encompass various aspects, such as nutrition, product choices, and lifestyle habits. By instilling these values early on, you can cultivate a sense of responsibility towards the planet in your child while also ensuring a healthier start to their life.

During pregnancy, mothers can adopt eco-friendly practices by focusing on nutrition and diet. Choosing organic and locally sourced foods not only supports sustainable farming practices but also minimizes exposure to harmful pesticides and chemicals, which is particularly critical during high-risk pregnancies. Prioritizing a diet rich in whole foods, fruits, and vegetables can contribute to both maternal health and fetal development. Moreover, involving your child in meal planning and preparation can enhance their understanding of where food comes from and the importance of making conscious food choices.

As your child grows, it is beneficial to introduce them to environmentally friendly products and practices. This can include using cloth diapers, eco-friendly toys, and natural cleaning supplies. Teaching your child about the importance of these choices can help them appreciate the impact of consumerism on the environment. Additionally, engaging in activities such as recycling, gardening, or participating in community clean-up events can foster a sense of connection to the earth. These experiences not only help children understand sustainability but also promote physical activity and mental well-being.

Educating your child about the environment can also extend to their understanding of cultural practices related to sustainability. Many cultures have traditions that emphasize harmony with nature, and sharing these stories can enrich your child's perspective. By incorporating cultural teachings about the environment, you can help them develop a deeper respect for diverse lifestyles and practices that honor the planet. Discussing the significance of these traditions can encourage critical thinking and empathy, reinforcing the idea that every action counts in protecting our world.

Finally, fostering an environmentally conscious mindset involves consistent communication and modeling of eco-friendly behaviors. As an expecting mother, your actions and attitudes can profoundly influence your child's views on the environment. Create opportunities for discussions about sustainability and involve them in making decisions that reflect these values. Whether it's choosing to walk or bike instead of driving, conserving water, or making mindful purchases, your active participation in eco-friendly practices can inspire your child to embrace a lifestyle that prioritizes the health of both themselves and the planet.

Chapter 9: Cultural Practices in Pregnancy

Understanding Diverse Traditions

The journey of pregnancy is not only a personal experience but also one deeply rooted in cultural traditions and practices that vary widely across different societies. Expecting mothers can benefit from exploring these diverse traditions as they can provide valuable insights into prenatal care, childbirth, and postpartum practices. Many cultures have unique rituals and beliefs that support women during pregnancy, encompassing aspects of nutrition, mental well-being, and community support. By understanding these traditions, mothers can make informed choices that resonate with their own values and enhance their pregnancy experience.

In various cultures, dietary practices during pregnancy are often guided by traditional beliefs about nutrition and health. For instance, some communities emphasize the consumption of specific foods thought to promote fetal health and maternal well-being. Foods rich in iron, calcium, and folate are frequently recommended, and certain herbs or spices may be believed to aid digestion or alleviate common pregnancy ailments. Expecting mothers can explore these cultural dietary practices to enrich their own nutritional plans, potentially incorporating beneficial foods that align with their health goals while respecting their cultural heritage.

Mental health during pregnancy is another aspect significantly influenced by cultural traditions. Many societies have established support systems where family, friends, and community members come together to support the expecting mother emotionally and spiritually. Rituals such as blessing ways or baby showers can create a sense of belonging and reduce feelings of isolation. Understanding these cultural practices can encourage mothers to seek out similar support networks, whether through family gatherings, community events, or online forums, thus fostering a supportive environment that prioritizes mental health during pregnancy.

Pregnancy after loss is a sensitive topic that intersects with cultural traditions as well. Many cultures have specific rituals to honor lost pregnancies and provide emotional support to mothers coping with grief. These practices can include memorial services, naming ceremonies, or family gatherings that acknowledge the loss while celebrating the hope of new beginnings. Engaging with these traditions can help expecting mothers process their emotions and find solace in shared experiences, allowing them to navigate their current pregnancy with greater resilience and understanding.

Finally, the cultural context surrounding pregnancy extends to workplace rights and the preparation of siblings for a new baby. Different cultures have varying expectations regarding maternity leave, workplace accommodations, and family dynamics. Additionally, traditions around introducing a new sibling can help children understand and adapt to the changes that come with a new addition to the family. By exploring these diverse cultural practices, expecting mothers can better advocate for their rights and prepare their families for the exciting journey ahead, ensuring a harmonious transition into parenthood.

Integrating Cultural Practices into Your Journey

Integrating cultural practices into your journey during a high-risk pregnancy can provide not only comfort but also a sense of connection to your heritage and community. Many cultures have long-standing traditions that emphasize the importance of support systems, nutrition, and mental well-being during pregnancy. Understanding and incorporating these practices can help you feel more empowered and connected to your pregnancy experience. It is essential to explore these traditions, as they can offer valuable insights and lessons that resonate with your unique situation.

Cultural practices often include specific dietary guidelines, rituals, and community support mechanisms that have been passed down through generations. For instance, many cultures emphasize the significance of consuming nutrient-dense foods that are believed to benefit both the mother and the growing baby. Engaging with these dietary practices can enhance your nutrition plan, ensuring that you receive essential vitamins and minerals, which are particularly important in high-risk pregnancies. Consider discussing these cultural dietary traditions with your healthcare provider to ensure they align with your medical needs.

Mental health is a critical aspect of navigating a high-risk pregnancy, and cultural practices can play a vital role in providing emotional support. Many cultures emphasize communal gatherings and sharing experiences with other mothers, which can alleviate feelings of isolation. Creating a supportive network through cultural groups or community organizations can help you connect with others who understand your journey. Engaging in cultural rituals, such as blessings or celebrations, can also foster a sense of belonging and reinforce a positive mindset during this challenging time.

Incorporating cultural practices into prenatal fitness and exercise routines is another way to enhance your pregnancy experience. Various cultures have unique approaches to physical activity during pregnancy, often rooted in traditional dances or movements that promote flexibility and strength. Finding a class or community group that focuses on these culturally relevant activities can make exercising more enjoyable and meaningful. Always consult with your healthcare provider to ensure that any physical activity you choose is safe for your specific circumstances.

Lastly, integrating cultural practices into your pregnancy journey can extend to preparing siblings for the arrival of a new baby. Many cultures have specific customs or storytelling traditions that help older children understand and embrace their new roles. Engaging siblings in these practices can ease the transition and foster a sense of responsibility and love. Discussing family traditions or creating new rituals centered around the baby's arrival can help siblings feel included and excited about the upcoming changes, reinforcing the importance of family support during this period.

Respecting Personal and Family Beliefs

Respecting personal and family beliefs is a fundamental aspect of navigating high-risk pregnancies. Expecting mothers often find themselves at the intersection of medical advice and personal values, making it essential to honor their individual beliefs while also considering the recommendations of healthcare professionals. Each pregnancy is unique, and personal beliefs can encompass a wide range of factors including cultural practices, religious traditions, and family values. Understanding and respecting these beliefs can significantly enhance the emotional well-being of the mother and foster a supportive environment during this vulnerable time.

Cultural practices play a vital role in shaping how individuals approach pregnancy and childbirth. Many expecting mothers may wish to incorporate traditional customs and rituals that align with their heritage. These practices can provide comfort and a sense of continuity, allowing mothers to connect with their family history. It is important for healthcare providers to engage in open dialogues with their patients about these cultural beliefs, ensuring that medical recommendations are sensitive to and compatible with personal values. This approach can help mitigate feelings of conflict and enhance the overall pregnancy experience.

Religious beliefs also significantly influence pregnancy choices, from dietary restrictions to the preferred method of childbirth. For instance, some mothers may prioritize natural childbirth based on their faith's teachings about the sanctity of life and the natural process of birth. Others may have specific dietary laws that they wish to adhere to during pregnancy. Healthcare professionals should approach these discussions with empathy and respect, offering support that aligns medical advice with the mother's spiritual beliefs. By doing so, they not only empower mothers but also build a trusting relationship that is crucial during high-risk pregnancies.

Mental health is another critical aspect that intersects with personal and family beliefs during pregnancy. Expecting mothers may experience anxiety or fear, particularly in high-risk situations. It is vital for them to feel supported in expressing their concerns and preferences regarding mental health care. Some may choose to seek therapy that aligns with their beliefs, such as faith-based counseling, while others might prefer more traditional therapeutic approaches. Encouraging mothers to discuss their preferences can facilitate tailored mental health support that respects their values, ultimately enhancing their emotional resilience.

Finally, workplace rights and family dynamics also play significant roles in how personal and family beliefs manifest during pregnancy. Expecting mothers often face challenges in balancing their professional responsibilities with their health and family needs. Understanding one's rights in the workplace, particularly regarding maternity leave and accommodations, is essential. Additionally, preparing siblings for a new baby can involve family traditions and beliefs, creating a harmonious environment as the family grows. By recognizing and respecting these beliefs, expecting mothers can navigate their pregnancies with confidence and assurance, knowing their values are honored throughout the journey.

Chapter 10: Pregnancy and Workplace Rights

Understanding Your Rights as an Expecting Mother

Understanding your rights as an expecting mother is crucial for ensuring a safe and supportive environment during your pregnancy. As you navigate the complexities of a high-risk pregnancy, it is essential to be aware of the legal protections and rights that are available to you. This knowledge can empower you to advocate for your health and well-being, as well as that of your unborn child. Familiarizing yourself with these rights can also help alleviate some of the stress that often accompanies high-risk pregnancies, allowing you to focus on your physical and mental health.

One of the most significant rights you have as an expecting mother is the right to receive comprehensive prenatal care. This includes access to healthcare providers who are knowledgeable about high-risk pregnancies and can offer personalized care plans tailored to your specific needs. You should feel empowered to ask questions, voice your concerns, and seek second opinions if necessary. Understanding your rights in relation to prenatal care can help ensure that you receive the best possible support throughout your pregnancy, which is particularly important when managing potential complications.

Your workplace rights during pregnancy are another critical aspect to consider. Under the Family and Medical Leave Act (FMLA) in the United States, eligible employees are entitled to take unpaid, job-protected leave for certain family and medical reasons, including pregnancy. This means that you have the right to take time off work to attend prenatal appointments or to recover after childbirth without fear of losing your job. Additionally, many employers are required to provide reasonable accommodations for pregnant employees, such as modified duties or flexible scheduling, to support your health and well-being during this time.

In terms of mental health, it is vital to recognize your right to access mental health resources during pregnancy. High-risk pregnancies can bring about heightened anxiety and emotional challenges, making it essential to seek support from professionals who specialize in maternal mental health. You have the right to discuss these concerns with your healthcare provider and to receive referrals to therapists or support groups if needed. Prioritizing your mental health is just as important as your physical health, and understanding your rights in this area can help you navigate the emotional complexities of pregnancy.

Lastly, consider the cultural practices surrounding pregnancy and the potential rights you have to incorporate those practices into your prenatal care. Many cultures have specific traditions and beliefs regarding pregnancy that can enhance your experience and provide comfort. You have the right to communicate these preferences to your healthcare provider and seek care that respects your cultural values. Embracing your cultural identity during pregnancy can foster a sense of connection and support, making your journey through a high-risk pregnancy more holistic and personally meaningful.

Navigating Maternity Leave

Maternity leave is an essential consideration for expecting mothers, especially those navigating high-risk pregnancies. Understanding the policies and options available can significantly reduce stress and ensure a smoother transition into motherhood. Most employers offer maternity leave, but the duration and conditions can vary widely. Familiarizing yourself with the Family and Medical Leave Act (FMLA) and your company's specific policies is crucial. This knowledge empowers you to plan ahead, ensuring you can take the necessary time off for both your health and the well-being of your newborn.

In high-risk pregnancies, the need for maternity leave may arise earlier than anticipated. Complications such as preeclampsia, gestational diabetes, or other medical concerns can necessitate extended time off work. It is essential to discuss your situation with your healthcare provider, who can give guidance on when to start your leave. Open communication with your employer about your medical needs is vital as well. Providing documentation from your healthcare provider can help in securing the leave you require.

Planning your maternity leave also involves considering how to effectively manage your workload before your departure. Creating a comprehensive transition plan can ensure that your responsibilities are adequately delegated during your absence. This may include detailed instructions for coworkers, setting clear expectations, and establishing a point of contact for urgent matters. By taking proactive steps, you can minimize stress for both yourself and your team, making your maternity leave more enjoyable and focused on your health and family.

Mental health is another critical aspect to keep in mind when navigating maternity leave. The transition to motherhood can bring about a range of emotions, from joy to anxiety. Ensuring that you have a support system in place, whether through family, friends, or mental health professionals, is essential. Taking time for self-care during your leave will help you adjust to the new changes in your life. Engaging in activities that promote mental well-being, such as prenatal yoga or mindfulness practices, can also be beneficial during this time.

Finally, considering the cultural aspects of maternity leave is important for many expecting mothers. Different cultures have varying approaches to maternity leave, and understanding these can help you find a balance that respects your background while accommodating your needs. Additionally, if you have older children, preparing them for the arrival of a new sibling during your leave can strengthen family bonds. Engage them in the process, involve them in discussions, and ensure they feel included in the transition. By thoughtfully navigating maternity leave, you set the stage for a positive experience as you embark on this new chapter of motherhood.

Communicating with Employers

Communicating with employers during a high-risk pregnancy is essential for ensuring both your well-being and job security. It is important to approach the conversation with clarity and confidence, as this will help you express your needs while also fostering understanding among your colleagues and supervisors. Start by scheduling a private meeting with your employer or HR representative to discuss your situation, ensuring that you have their full attention and can speak freely. Prepare for this meeting by gathering any necessary documentation from your healthcare provider that outlines your pregnancy status and any recommended accommodations.

When discussing your high-risk pregnancy with your employer, be open about your condition, focusing on how it may affect your work responsibilities. Clearly articulate any limitations or necessary adjustments, such as reduced hours, flexibility for medical appointments, or the option to work from home if feasible. It is vital to emphasize that you are committed to your role and want to ensure that your health remains a top priority, as well as the quality of your work. This approach not only demonstrates professionalism but also reinforces your dedication to your job.

Employers are often more receptive to accommodating employees when they are informed and engaged in the conversation. Be prepared to discuss potential solutions that could benefit both parties. For example, if your role allows, suggest delegating specific tasks to colleagues or adjusting deadlines to ensure that your workload remains manageable. Highlighting these options can make it easier for your employer to understand how they can support you while maintaining team productivity.

Understanding your workplace rights is crucial during this time. Familiarize yourself with local labor laws regarding pregnancy and maternity leave, as well as any company policies in place that protect your rights as a pregnant employee. If your employer is unresponsive or unsupportive, you may need to seek advice from a legal expert or a pregnancy support organization to ensure that you are treated fairly. Knowing your rights empowers you to advocate for yourself effectively and ensures that you receive the necessary accommodations during your high-risk pregnancy.

Finally, maintain open lines of communication throughout your pregnancy. Regular check-ins with your employer can help keep them updated on your condition and any changes in your needs. This ongoing dialogue fosters a collaborative relationship, allowing for adjustments as necessary while demonstrating your proactive approach. Remember, you are not alone in this journey; many women navigate high-risk pregnancies, and sharing your experiences can foster a supportive environment within your workplace.

Chapter 11: Preparing Siblings for a New Baby

Discussing the Pregnancy with Siblings

When discussing an impending pregnancy with siblings, it is essential to approach the topic with sensitivity and clarity. Siblings, especially younger ones, may have a limited understanding of what pregnancy entails and how it will affect their lives. Introducing the idea of a new family member should be framed positively, emphasizing the excitement and joy that a new baby brings. Use age-appropriate language and encourage open dialogue, allowing siblings to express their thoughts and feelings about the upcoming changes.

It's crucial to acknowledge and validate any feelings of uncertainty or jealousy that siblings may experience. These emotions are natural and can arise when a child senses their position within the family may change. Providing reassurance that love and attention will continue to be shared can help alleviate these concerns. Engaging siblings in the pregnancy journey can foster a sense of inclusion, making them feel important and valued. This can be done through simple activities, such as attending prenatal appointments or helping to prepare the nursery, which can help them feel more connected to the experience.

Encouraging siblings to participate in discussions about the baby's arrival can also promote a sense of responsibility and excitement. Involving them in planning for the baby's needs, such as selecting items for the nursery or picking out baby clothes, can ignite their imagination and enthusiasm. Moreover, discussing the baby's milestones and what they can expect when the baby arrives can help reduce anxiety. Providing siblings with books or resources about becoming an older sibling can further prepare them for this significant transition, ensuring they feel informed and engaged.

It is also vital to maintain some normalcy in siblings' lives during this period of change. Balancing attention between the new baby and existing children helps to prevent feelings of neglect. Establishing routines that incorporate one-on-one time with siblings can reinforce their importance in the family dynamic. Additionally, discussing how they can be involved in caring for the baby—whether through simple tasks like fetching diapers or singing to the baby—can create a nurturing environment that fosters sibling bonding.

Finally, keeping the lines of communication open throughout the pregnancy and after the baby's arrival is critical. Regularly checking in with siblings about their feelings and experiences can help them navigate any challenges that arise. As the family grows, encouraging discussions about their thoughts and feelings will support emotional well-being and strengthen family bonds. By fostering a supportive atmosphere, expecting mothers can help siblings embrace their new roles, ensuring a smoother transition for the entire family.

Involving Siblings in the Process

Involving siblings in the process of preparing for a new baby can be both enriching and beneficial for the entire family, especially in the context of high-risk pregnancies. As expecting mothers navigate the unique challenges associated with their situation, it is essential to consider how to engage older siblings in a way that fosters understanding, support, and excitement. By actively involving them in the journey, you can help mitigate feelings of jealousy or confusion, and instead promote a sense of belonging and responsibility toward the new family member.

One effective approach is to have open discussions about the pregnancy, tailored to the age and understanding of the siblings. This can include explaining the reasons behind the high-risk designation, utilizing age-appropriate language and concepts. For younger children, simple explanations can alleviate fears, while older siblings may appreciate more in-depth conversations about the medical aspects and potential outcomes. Providing a safe space for questions can encourage siblings to express their feelings and concerns, making them feel valued and included in the process.

In addition to communication, involving siblings in practical preparations can enhance their connection to the new baby. Activities such as decorating the nursery, choosing baby clothes, or selecting toys can create shared experiences that foster excitement. Additionally, involving them in discussions about prenatal nutrition and fitness can help them understand the importance of maternal health. For instance, allowing siblings to help prepare healthy meals or engage in family-friendly exercises can reinforce the idea that everyone plays a role in supporting the mother's well-being during this critical time.

Another important aspect is to address potential emotional responses that siblings may experience throughout the pregnancy. High-risk situations can create anxiety and uncertainty, not just for the expecting mother but for the whole family. It is crucial to validate any feelings of worry or fear that siblings may express. Encouraging them to share their emotions and providing reassurance can strengthen family bonds. Consider introducing activities such as family meetings or art projects that allow siblings to express their feelings creatively, fostering an environment where their thoughts and emotions are acknowledged.

Lastly, reinforcing the idea of family unity as the new baby arrives can help siblings transition smoothly into their new roles. This can be achieved by discussing the importance of helping and caring for the baby, emphasizing that they will always be an essential part of the family dynamic. Involving siblings in tasks such as diaper changes or holding the baby, under supervision, can build confidence and a sense of purpose. By ensuring that siblings feel included and appreciated, you are not only preparing them for the arrival of a new family member but also nurturing a loving and supportive family environment that is crucial, particularly in the context of a high-risk pregnancy.

Addressing Concerns and Emotions

Addressing concerns and emotions during a high-risk pregnancy is crucial for the overall well-being of both the mother and the developing baby. Expecting mothers may experience a range of emotions, from anxiety and fear to hope and excitement. Acknowledging these feelings is the first step toward managing them effectively. It is important to create an open environment where mothers can express their concerns without judgment. This encourages communication with healthcare providers, family members, and support networks, which can alleviate feelings of isolation and stress.

One common concern during high-risk pregnancies is the fear of complications that could arise. Expecting mothers may worry about the health of their baby, the potential for preterm labor, or the impact of their condition on their daily lives. Providing accurate information and education about specific risks associated with high-risk pregnancies can help demystify these fears. Engaging in discussions with healthcare professionals can empower mothers to make informed decisions, ultimately helping them feel more in control of their situation.

Mental health plays a significant role in managing a high-risk pregnancy. The emotional strain can lead to conditions such as anxiety and depression, which may affect both the mother and the baby. Incorporating strategies for mental wellness, such as mindfulness practices, yoga, and prenatal counseling, can help mothers navigate their emotional landscape. Finding a supportive community, whether through online forums or local support groups, can also provide a vital outlet for sharing experiences and receiving encouragement from others who understand their journey.

Nutrition and physical health are equally important when addressing emotional concerns during pregnancy. A well-balanced diet rich in essential nutrients can positively impact mood and energy levels. Expecting mothers should focus on foods that support both their mental and physical health. Additionally, prenatal fitness and exercise, tailored to a high-risk pregnancy, can enhance mood and reduce anxiety. Engaging in gentle activities, like walking or swimming, can promote relaxation and a sense of accomplishment, contributing to overall emotional well-being.

Finally, preparing siblings for the arrival of a new baby can also evoke a range of emotions. Ensuring that older children feel included and valued during this transition is essential. Open discussions about the changes they can expect, along with opportunities for them to be involved in preparations, can help alleviate feelings of jealousy or anxiety. By addressing these concerns and fostering a supportive family environment, mothers can help their children embrace the new addition with excitement and love. In summary, addressing concerns and emotions during a high-risk pregnancy involves creating a supportive atmosphere, focusing on mental and physical health, and preparing the entire family for the journey ahead.

Chapter 12: Resources and Support

Finding Support Groups

Finding support groups during a high-risk pregnancy can be an essential step for expecting mothers navigating the complexities of their situation. These groups provide a space where women can share experiences, exchange advice, and find comfort in knowing they are not alone. Engaging with others who understand the unique challenges of a high-risk pregnancy can significantly alleviate feelings of isolation and anxiety. Many hospitals, clinics, and community centers offer support groups specifically tailored for high-risk pregnancies, so it is beneficial to explore these local resources.

Online support groups have also become increasingly popular, providing 24/7 access to a network of women facing similar circumstances. Platforms like social media, forums, and dedicated websites can connect expecting mothers with others globally, allowing for diverse perspectives and shared experiences. These virtual communities often foster a sense of camaraderie and understanding, as members can discuss everything from prenatal fitness plans to coping strategies for managing mental health during pregnancy. Participating in these groups can empower women to make informed decisions about their pregnancy and childbirth.

When seeking out support groups, it is essential to consider the specific needs that resonate with you. Some groups may focus primarily on emotional support, while others might emphasize practical advice on nutrition and exercise tailored for high-risk pregnancies. Additionally, there are groups that address cultural practices and workplace rights, helping mothers navigate their unique circumstances. By identifying the areas where you need the most support, you can find the right group that aligns with your values and expectations.

In-person meetings often foster deeper connections among members, allowing for more meaningful conversations and friendships to develop. Look for local classes or workshops that cater to high-risk pregnancies, as these settings can also function as informal support groups. Engaging with healthcare professionals in these environments can offer invaluable insights into managing your pregnancy while also addressing any concerns regarding natural childbirth or prenatal care. Having a supportive community can make a significant difference in your overall pregnancy experience.

Finally, it is important to remember that seeking support is a sign of strength, not weakness. Whether through formal groups, online communities, or informal gatherings with friends and family, finding a network of support can lead to improved mental health and a more positive pregnancy experience. These connections can also extend beyond pregnancy, providing lasting relationships and continued support as you transition into motherhood. Prioritizing your emotional and physical well-being during this time is crucial, and finding the right support group can be a pivotal step in your journey.

Recommended Books and Websites

For expecting mothers navigating high-risk pregnancies, having access to reliable information is crucial. A variety of books and websites can provide valuable insights and guidance on managing the complexities of pregnancy. Notable titles such as "The Pregnancy Handbook for Couples" by Dr. Anne Deans offer practical advice tailored to both partners, emphasizing communication and support during high-risk situations. Another essential read is "Expecting Better" by Emily Oster, which combines personal anecdotes with data-driven insights, allowing mothers to make informed decisions regarding their health and pregnancy choices.

In the realm of natural childbirth preparation, "The Birth Partner" by Penny Simkin is a comprehensive resource that equips partners with the knowledge and skills necessary to support the birthing process effectively. This book covers various scenarios that may arise during labor, especially in high-risk cases, and offers strategies for emotional and physical support. Additionally, "Natural Childbirth the Bradley Way" provides a detailed approach to preparing for a natural birth, emphasizing the importance of prenatal education and fitness.

Nutrition plays a pivotal role in the health of both mother and baby, particularly in high-risk pregnancies. "Real Food for Pregnancy" by Lily Nichols offers a research-based approach to prenatal nutrition, focusing on whole foods and their impact on fetal development. This book provides meal plans and recipes, making it easier for mothers to integrate healthy eating into their daily lives. For those seeking plant-based options, "The Vegan Pregnancy Cookbook" by Vegan Family Kitchen presents nutritious, easy-to-follow recipes tailored for expecting mothers aiming for a balanced diet.

Mental health is another vital aspect during high-risk pregnancies, and "The Mindful Way Through Pregnancy" by Susan M. Pollak focuses on cultivating mindfulness to reduce anxiety and promote emotional well-being. This book offers practical exercises and meditative practices designed to help mothers cope with the stresses of pregnancy. Complementing this, websites like Postpartum Support International provide valuable resources and community support for mothers experiencing mental health challenges, ensuring they have access to the help they need.

Finally, understanding workplace rights during pregnancy is essential for expecting mothers. The website of the U.S. Equal Employment Opportunity Commission offers comprehensive information on pregnancy discrimination and rights in the workplace, empowering mothers to advocate for themselves. For those interested in eco-friendly pregnancy and parenting, "The Green Baby Handbook" serves as a guide to sustainable choices throughout pregnancy and beyond. These resources, alongside culturally relevant practices found in books like "The Spiritual Woman's Guide to Pregnancy," can help mothers navigate their unique journeys with confidence and knowledge.

Healthcare Resources for High-Risk Pregnancies

Healthcare resources for high-risk pregnancies encompass a variety of services and support systems designed to ensure the health and well-being of both the mother and the baby. Expecting mothers identified as being at high risk due to factors such as age, medical history, or pregnancy complications can benefit greatly from accessing specialized healthcare resources. Hospitals often have maternal-fetal medicine specialists who focus on high-risk pregnancies and can provide tailored care plans. Regular consultations with these specialists can help monitor the pregnancy, address any complications early, and provide the necessary interventions to promote a healthy outcome.

In addition to specialized medical care, expecting mothers should consider utilizing support groups and educational programs that focus on high-risk pregnancies. Many healthcare facilities and community organizations offer workshops and seminars aimed at educating women about their specific risks and the best practices for managing them. These programs often cover topics such as prenatal nutrition, exercise, and mental health, empowering mothers to take an active role in their care. Connecting with other mothers in similar situations can also provide emotional support and practical advice, creating a sense of community during a challenging time.

Prenatal care is critical for high-risk pregnancies, and it involves more frequent monitoring and check-ups compared to low-risk pregnancies. Expecting mothers should be proactive in scheduling regular appointments, which may include ultrasounds, blood tests, and other diagnostic procedures. These visits not only help to track the baby's development but also allow healthcare providers to detect potential issues early on. Being informed about what to expect during these appointments can help mothers feel more prepared and engaged in their pregnancy journey.

Nutrition and diet play a vital role in the management of high-risk pregnancies. Healthcare providers often recommend specific dietary guidelines that can help mitigate risks associated with gestational diabetes, hypertension, or other pregnancy-related conditions. Expecting mothers should focus on a balanced diet rich in whole foods, including fruits, vegetables, whole grains, lean proteins, and healthy fats. Consulting with a registered dietitian who specializes in prenatal nutrition can provide personalized meal plans and guidance tailored to individual health needs and preferences.

Mental health is another crucial aspect of navigating high-risk pregnancies. The emotional toll of potential complications can lead to increased anxiety and stress, so it is essential for mothers to prioritize their mental well-being. Accessing mental health resources, such as counseling or therapy, can provide valuable support. Additionally, practicing mindfulness techniques, engaging in prenatal fitness activities, and establishing a support network can help manage stress levels. By addressing both physical and mental health, expecting mothers can foster a healthier environment for themselves and their babies.

www.ingramcontent.com/pod-product-compliance
Lightning Source LLC
Chambersburg PA
CBHW072251260726
48657CB00005BA/2048